Carb Cycling

The Simple Way to Work With Your Body to Burn Fat & Build Muscle

Thomas Rohmer

Copyright © 2017
Rohmerfitness All rights reserved.

No part of this publication may be reproduced, distributed, or transmitted in any form or by any means, including photocopying, recording, or other electronic or mechanical methods, without the prior written permission and consent of the publisher, except in the in the case of brief quotations embodied in product reviews and certain other non-commercial uses permitted by copyright law.

Disclaimer:

This guide has been created for informational and reference purposes only. The author, publisher, and any other affiliated parties cannot be held in any way accountable for any personal injuries or damage allegedly resulting from the information contained herein, or from any misuse of such guidance. Although strict measures have been taken to provide accurate information, the parties involved with the creation and publication of this guide take no responsibility for any issues that many arise from alleged discrepancies contained herein. It is strongly recommended that you consult a physician, personal trainer, and nutritionist prior to commencing this or any other workout or diet plan. This guide is not a substitute for professional personal guidance from a qualified medical professional. If you feel pain or discomfort at any point during exercises contained herein, cease the activity immediately and seek medical guidance.

Table of Contents

Chapter 1: Not All Carbs Are Created Equally..........6
Chapter 2: The Science Behind How Carb Cycling Works..12
Chapter 3: How to Set Up Your Own Carb Cycling Diet...15
Chapter 4: Macro Percentages for High and Low Carb Days..19
Chapter 5: Carb Cycling and Building Muscle........25
Chapter 6: Muscle Building Workout With Carb Cycling...33
Chapter 7: What About Cardio?...........................39
Chapter 8: 30 Low-Carb Recipes..........................44
Chapter 9: 15 High-Carb Recipes.........................79
Chapter 10: How to Track Your Calories and Macros...99
Chapter 11: Frequently Asked Questions.............102

Introduction:

Dieting is hard. Millions of people go on a diet every year, but most will fail to successfully lose weight and keep it off. And it makes sense as to why so few people are successful when trying to get fit. See if you can relate to a story similar to this:

1. You start a new diet.
2. Everything is smooth sailing for the first few weeks and you lose some weight.
3. Eventually, your metabolism slows down, and weight loss comes to a grinding halt.
4. In a desperate attempt to get back on track, you further restrict your calories.
5. You start to go insane because you're eating too few calories.
6. You quit, binge eat, and feel guilty about yourself for quitting.
7. A week or two later, after you've gotten over your latest incident, you decide to go at it again, and the vicious cycle repeats itself.

Luckily, there's a way you can escape this diet trap, and it's called carb cycling. Think of it this way—to get from point A to point B when driving a car, you'll need to use multiple tools: the steering wheel, gas pedal, brakes, etc. to get where you want to go. Most diets only use the gas pedal. It's go, go, go all of the time until you crash and burn.

It's insane to think you'll get anywhere only using the gas pedal of a car! However, with carb cycling, you'll strategically learn how and when to hit the brakes. This'll give your body a chance to recuperate and even further accelerate fat loss!

If that's something you're interested in then you're in the right place. This book will teach you everything you need to know about carb cycling: the science behind it, how to start your own carb cycling diet, and low carb/high carb recipes. Let's jump right in...

Chapter 1: Not All Carbs Are Created Equally

It's first important to understand exactly what carbs are and what their functions are in the body before we get into the ins and outs of carb cycling. Of the three macronutrients: protein, carbs and fat—carbohydrates are your body's first source of energy. Your body will burn off carbohydrates when you exercise to give you the necessary energy to complete the workout. They're also important for serotonin levels in the brain and proper nervous system functioning (1).

Without carbs, your body will soon start to run out of energy and you'll become irritable. If you've ever gone on a low carb diet, you've probably experienced this. For that reason alone, I don't advise going on a low carb diet as a long-term weight loss solution. To clarify, carb cycling isn't a low carb diet.

With carb cycling, you'll strategically have high and low carb days to change things up for continual fat loss. But don't worry about that now, I'll thoroughly explain everything about carb cycling in later chapters. For right now, you need to understand carbs and the differences between simple and complex carbs.

Is a Carbohydrate a Carbohydrate?

Many people love to debate about whether or not a calorie is a calorie. If I eat 100 calories from a cookie and you eat 100 calories from vegetables, are we equal? Well kinda.

One calorie *is* one calorie regardless of what source the calorie came from. Trying to argue with this is like saying one yard of wood isn't the same length as one yard of metal. The difference lies in the *macronutrient* quality.

100 calories from vegetables and 100 calories from a cookie are still 100 calories. Both are made up mostly of carbs; the quality of those carbs is what makes them very different. The cookie contains simple carbs and sugar.

It won't provide you with any vitamins, nutrients, or fiber. It also won't be very satiating. The vegetables, on the other hand, are complex carbs.

They'll provide you with quality complex carbs and a good source of vitamins, nutrients and fiber. Additionally, nutritious foods like fruits and vegetables will keep you fuller longer, which is critical during calorie restriction for weight loss purposes. Therefore, quality of calories can be as important as quantity of calories.

As you can tell, if you eat a low amount of carbs, but the quality of those carbs are poor in nutritional value then you'll still fail. You must eat the right kind of carbohydrates and in the right amounts in order to be successful.

Difference between Simple and Complex Carbohydrates

Many people define simple carbohydrates as carbs that contain sugar and complex carbohydrates as carbs that contain starch and fiber. However, this isn't fully true. Fruit contains sugar, but it's not a simple carbohydrate because it's natural sugar has a different effect on the body than added sugar contained in sodas and processed foods. Not only that, but some starch foods contain refined wheat flour and could cause health issues.

Here's a better way to define complex and simple carbohydrates:

Simple carbs: starches and sugars that have been refined and stripped of their natural nutrients and fiber.

Complex carbs: carbs found in whole, unprocessed foods such as fruits, vegetables, legumes and whole grains.

The main difference between complex and simple carbs is that complex carbs are nutrient dense; this means they contain a large amount of nutrients in relation to the total number of calories they provide. These carbs are rich in fiber, vitamins, minerals and antioxidants. Simple carbs, on the other hand, contain empty calories. They provide little to no nutritional value. Sure they may taste good, but they'll do little to keep you full, which is critical when your calories are restricted.

Health Benefits of Complex Carbs

Eating complex carbs can provide you with the following health benefits:

Fewer Blood Sugar Spikes:

Complex carbs take a longer time to digest, which means that your blood sugar won't spike like it would when you consume simple carbs. When your blood sugar levels increase, your body will release more insulin to digest the incoming carbs. This then leads to a blood sugar crash, which will leave you hungry and craving additional sugar (2).

Potential Reduction in Risk of Developing Chronic Diseases

Antioxidants, fiber, vitamins and minerals are all necessary for preventing disease. By consuming complex carbohydrates, you'll get an adequate dose of all of these, which can reduce you risk for developing certain diseases like diabetes and heart disease (3).

Healthier Digestive Track

Complex carbs contain more beneficial bacteria in them than simple carbs do. This bacteria will help digestive issues from occurring in your gut (4).

Inflammation Reduction:

Long-term inflammation can increase the risk for developing severe diseases. Simple carbs stimulate inflammation, while complex carbs work to reduce inflammation in the body (5).

Dangers of Simple Carbs:

Eating too many simple carbs can be harmful to your health over time. Here are some of the hazards of simple carbs:

They're Easy to Overeat:

Simple carbs are empty calories, which means that they won't satiate you. This'll make it easier to overeat on other foods so you can get full from your meal.

Increased Risk of Disease:

People who consume more sugar and processed foods are more likely to develop heart disease and type 2 diabetes than those who don't (6).

Sugar is Addicting:

There's research to show how addicting sugar can be. Some studies show that sugar can be just as addictive as drugs like cocaine because both cause the brain to release dopamine and stimulate the pleasure centers of our brains (7).

List of High Quality Complex Carbs to Consume in Your Diet

The following is a non-comprehensive list of complex carbs that you should consider eating in your diet on a regular basis:

- Whole Grain Oats
- Quinoa
- Brown rice
- Whole grain barley
- Black beans
- Kidney beans
- Black-eyed peas
- Sweet potatoes
- Chia seeds
- Flax seeds
- Any fruits
- Any green vegetables

List of Simple Carbs to Avoid or Eat Sparingly

The following is a non-comprehensive list of simple carbs that you should avoid eating or only eat in moderation:

- Sodas or beverages that contain excess calories or sugar
- Sweets and pastries such as cake, ice cream, candy, donuts, pop-tarts, etc.
- White bread
- White pastas

Hopefully you now understand the difference between simple and complex carbohydrates, and you can now clearly see that not all carbs are the same. My goal isn't to scare you into never eating any more refined carbs, but I want you to realize the importance of complex carbs. They're going to be critical for your success with carb cycling.

Chapter 2: The Science Behind How Carb Cycling Works

As I mentioned earlier, most diets fail because they only know how to hit the gas pedal and go, go, go. With carb cycling, you're going to go, go, and then hit the breaks and slow down for a bit before putting your foot back on the gas pedal.

When you restrict your caloric intake for a prolonged period of time to lose weight, your leptin levels will decrease. And as you're about to find out, this is a very important hormone for fat loss.

What is Leptin and Why Does it Matter?

Leptin is commonly referred to as the starvation hormone because its main job in the body is to regulate energy balance. At optimal levels, it tells the brain that we have enough fat stored, that we can stop eating and that we can continue burning calories at a normal pace. Essentially, leptin is there to prevent us from starving or overeating. In the hunter and gatherer days, this mechanism was essential for our survival.

Back then, calories were scarce and people didn't know when or where their next meal would come from. During times of food scarcity, leptin would kick in and slow down the person's metabolism and hold onto any fat stores that it could so they could be used at a later time. Fast-forward to the present day and things are much different.

Today, we live in a world with an overabundance of food. You can easily drive to the supermarket or a fast-food restaurant and get food 24/7. Although leptin was necessary for humans to survive this long, it can kind of be a pain-in-the-neck today. Consciously, you know you have access to food whenever you want it, but your body is still in the dark. That's why when you've got your diet down and things are going great, leptin will come in to crash the party. It still thinks you're starving and that food supply is low.

This is how leptin works in the body:

1. We eat
2. Body fat increases
3. Leptin levels increase
4. We eat less and burn more

Or:

1. We don't eat
2. Body fat decreases
3. Leptin levels decrease
4. We eat more and burn less

This is a classic case of "damned if you do, damned if you don't." On one hand, you can eat less, but as soon as you do, your leptin levels will decrease and you'll feel hungry, your appetite will increase and your motivation to exercise will decrease. On the other hand, you can eat more, which will decrease hunger, decrease appetite and increase motivation to workout. Unfortunately though, you're eating more and that's counterproductive to losing weight.

Break the Cycle With Another Cycle

The perfect solution to this catch-22 as you can probably guess is carb cycling. On your low-carb days, your body will be releasing low amounts of insulin, which will allow you to burn more fat. This is because your body doesn't burn off fat when your insulin levels are high; it'll be too busy burning off carbs instead. Of course, having low-carb days will start to decrease your leptin levels.

That's why you'll then have a high-carb day to offset the lowered leptin levels and get them back to normal. Once they're reset, you'll go back to your low-carb days and start burning fat again. You'll change things up at the right moment to trick your body and keep it guessing. You'll never give it the chance to catch onto what you're doing.

The high-carb days will also be beneficial for preserving your body's lean muscle mass. This is true for a couple of reasons:

1. Your glycogen stores will be replenished on your high-carbs, which will help keep your muscle cells full.

2. Your body is more likely to use muscle mass for energy when calories are restricted for extended periods of time (8).

Not only that, but cycling in high carb days will help you keep your sanity and allow you to sustain the diet. When things get hard, we give up and quit. It's much easier to keep going if you know that you're one day away from getting to consume a high amount of carbs again. However, with most diets, you have nothing to look forward to except for more misery. This is what makes having nothing but low-carb days tough, and that's why most people fail with a typical low-carb diet.

Now that you understand how carb cycling is effective, let's get started setting up your own carb cycling diet...

Chapter 3: How to Set Up Your Own Carb Cycling Diet

There are many different ways to set up a carb cycling diet. However, this is the most effective way to go about it:

Monday: Low-carb day
Tuesday: Low-carb day
Wednesday: Low-carb day
Thursday: High-carb day
Friday: Low-carb day
Saturday: Low-carb day
Sunday: Low-carb day
Following Monday: High-carb day

Essentially, you'll have 3 low-carb days in a row and then follow it with a high-carb day. Of course, you don't have to set up your schedule exactly like the example above. You could start your schedule out to where you have a high-carb day on a Saturday for example.

You can also change things around a bit to be more flexible with your schedule so that you eat high-carbs on a day you actually want to. For example, you might have 2 low-carb days in a row, have a high-carb day, and then go 4 days in a row eating a low amount of carbs. You want to have some wiggle room with the diet to make it easier to stick to.

And here's the step-by-step process you need to take to complete your carb cycling diet:

Step #1: Determine Your Total Daily Energy Expenditure (TDEE)

Your TDEE is simply the total number of calories you burn off in a given day. Figuring out your TDEE is the first and most important step in setting up your carb cycling diet. If you don't know your TDEE, you'll be guessing and hoping that you see results. You'll have no idea if you're overeating or eating too few calories.

And in case you're not aware, the following is how your body works in regards to weight loss/gain.

- If you eat more calories than your TDEE, you will gain weight.
- If you eat less calories than your TDEE, you will lose weight.
- If you eat right at your TDEE, then you will neither gain nor lose weight.

Since we're interested in losing weight, we're going to want to eat less than our TDEE. So how do you figure out your TDEE? There are many different equations to determine your TDEE. Regardless of what method you use to find your TDEE, it'll likely be off by 100-200 calories.

For an exact, accurate number, you would have to go to a lab and pay for a test to get it measured. Fortunately, you don't have to waste your time or money doing that. The formulas will be close enough for you to get results. I keep things simple, and this is the formula you'll use to determine your TDEE:

Bodyweight (in pounds) x 13=TDEE

Using myself as an example:

Bodyweight 200 pounds x 13= 2,600 calories

This means:

If I eat more than 2,600 calories per day, I'll start to gain weight.
If I eat less than 2,600 calories per day, I'll start to lose weight.
If I eat 2,600 calories per day, I'll neither gain nor lose weight.

It's pretty simple, right? Sadly, most people have no clue how many calories they're burning off in a given day. And they don't know that they need to eat below their TDEE to start losing weight. They'll blindly start eating healthy and hope for the best. By learning this information, you put yourself ahead of 95% of people who are looking to lose weight.

Step #2: Set Up Your Macros for Low-Carb Days

Carbs are going to make up 20% of your total calories on low-carb days. Full details will be provided for setting up your macros in chapter 4.

Step #3: Set Up Your Macros for High-Carb Days

Carbs will make-up 50% of your total calories on high-carb days. Again, refer to chapter 4 for full details on setting up your macro percentages.

Step #4: Accurately Track and Record Your Calories and Macros

With carb cycling, you want to be as precise as possible with your caloric intake. You can't guess at how many calories certain foods contain. What gets measured gets managed, and in chapter 10, I'll share with you how you can easily and precisely track your calories and macros.

Step #5: Monitor and Adjust Accordingly

Along the way, you might find that you were measuring something wrong or you need to change something. With this step, you'll only make adjustments when necessary. For example, if you go two weeks in a row without losing weight, you'll need to assess and identify what's getting miscalculated so it can be fixed.

Chapter 4: Macro Percentages for High and Low Carb Days

If you're unaware, a macro is short for macronutrient, and they're basically nutrients that provide the body with energy. The body then uses this energy to carry out all of its processes: breathing, organ function, digestion, moving and a whole lot more. There are three macronutrients: protein, carbohydrates and fat. All three macronutrients have their own importance and are essential for survival.

Protein is the body's building block for things like muscle, hair, bones and skin. Fat acts as an insulator for the body, helps maintain normal body temperature and it's used as an energy source when carb stores are low. And as I mentioned earlier, carbs are your body's first source of energy, and they're important for serotonin levels in the brain and proper nervous system functioning.

Macronutrients shouldn't be confused with micronutrients. Micronutrients are nutrients needed in trace amounts for normal growth and development in living organisms. They include things such as vitamins and minerals. However, our main concern with this chapter will be focused on macronutrients. Specifically, the amounts of each macro needed to reach our fitness goals. Before we get into the specific macro percentages, it's important to know the following:

- 1 gram of protein contains 4 calories
- 1 gram of carbohydrate contains 4 calories
- 1 gram of fat contains 9 calories

Knowing this information will help you track the total amount of calories you're consuming for each macronutrient.

Macronutrients for Low-Carb Days

Consume the following macros and calories during your low-carb days:

- **Total calories:** Consume 25% less calories than your total daily energy expenditure (TDEE)
- **Protein:** 1 gram per pound of bodyweight
- **Carbs:** 20% of total calories
- **Fat:** Remaining calories after protein and carbs

I'll use myself as an example for determining the calculations:

As a reminder, calculate your TDEE by multiplying your bodyweight by 13.

Bodyweight=200 x 13= TDEE of 2,600 calories

TDEE on low-carb days:

2,600 x .25= 650

2,600-650=1,950 total daily calories on low-carb days

Protein on low-carb days:

Your protein intake on low-carb days will simply be 1 gram of protein per pound of bodyweight:

1 gram per pound of bodyweight= 200 daily grams of protein

4 calories in 1 gram of protein x 200= 800 total calories from protein

Carbs on low-carb days:

To determine your carb intake on low-carb days, take your TDEE on low-carb days and multiply it by .2:

1,950 x .2= 390 total calories from carbs

You can then divide that number by 4 to get the gram equivalent:

390/4= 97.5 grams of carbs per day

Fat on low-carb days:

Your remaining calories will come from fat. Take your calculated TDEE, subtract your protein and carb calories from that number, and you'll be left with your calories from fat:

1,950 (TDEE)-800 (protein)-390 (carbs)=760 total calories from fat

You can then divide this number by 9 to get the gram equivalent:

760/9= 84.4 grams of fat per day

In summary, this would be my macros and calories on a low-carb day:

TDEE=1,950 calories
Protein= 200 grams (800 calories)
Carbs= 97.5 grams (390 calories)
Fat= 84.4 grams (760 calories)

Macronutrients for High-Carb Days

Consume the following macros and calories on your high-carb days:

- Total calories: Consume 10% less calories than your total daily energy expenditure.
- Protein: 1 gram per pound of bodyweight

- Carbs: 50% of total calories
- Fat: Remaining calories after protein and carbs

I'll use myself as an example again for determining the calculations:

TDEE on high-carb days:

2,600 x .10= 260

2,600-260=2,340 total calories on high-carb days

Protein on high-carb days:

Your protein intake on high-carb days will simply be 1 gram of protein per pound of bodyweight:

1 gram per pound of bodyweight= 200 daily grams of protein

4 calories in 1 gram of protein x 200= 800 total calories from protein

Carbs on high-carb days:

To determine your carb intake on high-carb days, take your TDEE on high-carb days and multiply it by .5:

2,340 x .5= 1,170 total calories from carbs

You can then divide that number by 4 to get the gram equivalent:

1,170/4= 292.5 grams of carbs per day

Fat on high-carb days:

Your remaining calories will come from fat. Take your calculated TDEE, subtract your protein and carb calories from that number, and you'll be left with your calories from fat:

2,340 (TDEE)-800 (protein)-1,170 (carbs)=370 total calories from fat

You can then divide this number by 9 to get the gram equivalent:

370/9= 41.1 grams of fat per day

In summary, this would be my macros and calories on a high-carb day:

TDEE=2,340 calories
Protein= 200 grams (800 calories)
Carbs= 292.5 grams (1,170 calories)
Fat= 41.1 grams (370 calories)

You might be wondering why we're still eating 20% of our total calories from carbs on low-carb days. The reason why is because this is a low-carb day, not a no-carb day. Recall that carbs have many useful functions, and they're still making up a small percentage of the overall calories. It's high enough for you to keep your sanity (so you won't quit on the diet), but low enough for it to still be effective.

Then on your high-carb days, you're increasing your carb intake by *30%*—that's a big jump! It's definitely enough of a difference for your body to replenish leptin levels, which is exactly what we want. Going from 0% carbs to 50% would be too big of a leap, but a 30% increase hits the sweet spot.

You might also be wondering about protein. Why so much of it regardless of whether it's a high or low-carb day? You're consuming one gram of protein per pound of bodyweight for a couple of reasons:

#1: Protein has the highest thermic effect of food (TEF) of all 3 macronutrients.

The thermic effect of food is simply the amount of energy required to eat, digest, absorb and store food. Essentially, your body burns calories to digest the foods you eat!

Here's the approximate TEF for each macronutrient:

- Protein: 30-35%
- Carbs: 5-15%
- Fat: 3-4%

This means that if you consume 100 calories from protein, your body will burn roughly 30-35 calories to digest and process those original 100 calories. Conversely, if you consumed 100 calories from carbs, your body would only burn about 5-15 calories to digest and process the original 100 calories.

And since your calories are being restricted, it makes sense to consume high amounts of protein to maximize the TEF effect.

#2: Eating too little of protein when calories are restricted can lead to muscle loss

As you learned earlier, when you lower your calories for a prolonged period of time, your body will respond by slowing down your metabolism and holding onto body fat. Your body will still need energy to survive and function, so it'll get it by other means—i.e. your muscle mass. Fortunately, protein has a muscle-sparring effect (9), so if you consume enough of it, you'll be able to retain your lean muscle mass while dieting down. It won't do you any good to lose 20 pounds if 10 of those lost pounds were muscle.

Chapter 5: Carb Cycling and Building Muscle

Thus far, I've only talked about how you can use carb cycling as a way to lean down while retaining muscle mass. But what if your fitness goal is to build muscle? Can you still use carb cycling as a nutritional strategy to get the job done? The answer is yes, of course you can!

Carb cycling will make it easier for you to build muscle and at the same time minimize fat gain. It won't do you any good to bulk up and add 20 pounds to your frame if half of that weight is fat. You'll have to spend more time later cutting the fat you gained from the bulk!

What Changes When You Want to Build Muscle Instead of Burn Fat?

In terms of nutrition, the main thing that'll change when you want to build muscle is the amount of calories you eat. When your goal is to lose weight, you'll want to eat less calories than your total daily energy expenditure. When you want to build muscle, you'll want to consume more calories than your total daily energy expenditure. Calories are the building blocks your body will use to pack on lean muscle. Without enough calories, it won't be able to get the job done.

Think of it this way. Let's say you're a fisherman who wants to catch 100 fish in your net at a time. In order to do that, you'll need a net that's big enough to hold 100 fish in it. If your net can only hold 75 fish at a time then it won't be possible for you to reach your goal.

The same goes for calories and building muscle. For example, let's say your body needs 2,800 calories a day in order to build muscle. If you only eat 2,600 calories a day, then you're leaving muscle on the table because you're shorting your body of the necessary energy it needs to complete the task.

How Many Calories Do I Need to Eat to Start Building Muscle?

The key with calories and building muscle is to eat enough for your body to add mass, but not too much to where your body will store the excess calories as fat. You can't eat more and more and gain muscle in proportion to how much you're eating! Your body will use what it needs and then it'll store the rest as fat. That's why we want to eat right at that threshold where we'll add muscle but little to no fat.

To do that, we'll simply add 10% more calories to our total daily energy expenditure (TDEE).

Here's how to calculate it using myself as an example:

- 13 x bodyweight (200 pounds in my case)= TDEE of 2,600 calories
- 2,600 x .10= 260
- 260+2,600=2,860 total calories

This means that I'll need to eat 2,860 calories a day to build muscle with minimal fat gain.

Setting Up Your Carb Cycling Schedule

For fat loss, it's ideal to have a 3:1 low/high-carb ratio to maximize results. That is, for every 3 days you eat low-carbs, you'll have 1 day of high-carbs. To build muscle, we're going to change things up a bit. You're going to use a 3:2 low/high-carb ratio. For every 3 days you eat low-carbs, you'll have 2 days of eating high-carbs. The cool thing is that you don't have to do all of your low and high-carb days lined up in row, all though you can do that if you like.

Here are some different ways to set up your carb cycling schedule to build lean muscle mass:

Option #1:

- Monday: Low-carb day
- Tuesday: Low-carb day
- Wednesday: Low-carb day
- Thursday: High-carb day
- Friday: High-carb day
- Saturday: Low-carb day
- Sunday: Low-carb day
- Following Monday: Low-carb day, etc.

Option #2:

- Monday: High-carb day
- Tuesday: Low-carb day
- Wednesday: High-carb day
- Thursday: Low-carb day
- Friday: Low-carb day
- Saturday: High-carb day
- Sunday: Low-carb day
- Following Monday: High-carb day
- Following Tuesday: Low-carb day
- Following Wednesday: Low-carb day, etc.

Essentially with option #2, you'll have one high-carb day, one low-carb day, one high-carb day, 2 low-carb days, and then you'll repeat the cycle.

If you're having trouble determining what option you want to use for your cycle, consider your workout schedule (don't worry I'll cover a solid workout routine in chapter 6 if you need help with that). Ideally, you would want to have high-carb days on the same days that you workout. This is because on workout days your body will be burning more calories, and it'll need the extra carbs to help fuel the workout and start the recovery process.

On your rest days, you'll be burning less overall calories, and thus the carbs won't be needed as much. Of course, you won't always be able to time it to where you workout on the same day as a high-carb day, but you'll want to align it up as much as you can.

Macro Percentages for High and Low-Carb Days

These calculations won't be too much different from the ones we used when the goal was weight loss. The two main differences are that you'll be consuming a higher percentage of your calories from carbs and that you'll be eating more total calories.

Macro Percentages for Low-Carb Days to Build Muscle

Consume the following macros and calories during your low-carb days to build muscle:

- Total calories: Consume 10% more calories than your total daily energy expenditure (TDEE)
- Protein: 1 gram per pound of bodyweight
- Carbs: 25% of total calories

- Fat: Remaining calories after protein and carbs

I'll use myself as an example for determining the calculations:

TDEE on low-carb days:

2,600 x .10= 260

2,600+260=2,860 total daily calories on low-carb days

Protein on low-carb days:

Your protein intake on low-carb days will simply be 1 gram of protein per pound of bodyweight:

1 gram per pound of bodyweight= 200 daily grams of protein

4 calories in 1 gram of protein x 200= 800 total calories from protein

Carbs on low-carb days:

To determine your carb intake on low-carb days, take your TDEE on low-carb days and multiply it by .25:

2,860 x .25= 715 total calories from carbs

You can then divide that number by 4 to get the gram equivalent:

715/4= 178.75 grams of carbs per day

Fat on low-carb days:

Your remaining calories will come from fat. Take your calculated TDEE, subtract your protein and carb calories from that number, and you'll be left with your calories from fat:

2,860 (TDEE)-800 (protein)-715 (carbs)=1,345 total calories from fat

You can then divide this number by 9 to get the gram equivalent:

1,345/9= 149.4 grams of fat per day

In summary, this would be my macros and calories on a low-carb day to build muscle:

TDEE=2,860 calories
Protein= 200 grams (800 calories)
Carbs= 178.75 grams (715 calories)
Fat= 149.4 grams (1,345 calories)

Macro Percentages for High-Carb Days to Build Muscle

Consume the following macros and calories on your high-carb days to build muscle:

- Total calories: Consume 10% more calories than your total daily energy expenditure (TDEE). And yes, this means your TDEE will be the same on low and high-carb days!
- Protein: 1 gram per pound of bodyweight
- Carbs: 50% of total calories
- Fat: Remaining calories after protein and carbs

I'll use myself as an example again for determining the calculations:

TDEE on high-carb days:

2,600 x .10= 260

2,600+260=2,860 total calories on high-carb days

Protein on high-carb days:

Your protein intake on high-carb days will simply be 1 gram of protein per pound of bodyweight:

1 gram per pound of bodyweight= 200 daily grams of protein

4 calories in 1 gram of protein x 200= 800 total calories from protein

Carbs on high-carb days:

To determine your carb intake on high-carb days, take your TDEE on high-carb days and multiply it by .5:

2,860 x .50= 1,430 total calories from carbs

You can then divide that number by 4 to get the gram equivalent:

1,430/4= 357.5 grams of carbs per day

Fat on high-carb days:

Your remaining calories will come from fat. Take your calculated TDEE, subtract your protein and carb calories from that number, and you'll be left with your calories from fat:

2,860 (TDEE)-800 (protein)-1,430 (carbs)=630 total calories from fat

You can then divide this number by 9 to get the gram equivalent:

630/9= 70 grams of fat per day

In summary, this would be my macros and calories on a high-carb day:

TDEE=2,860 calories
Protein= 200 grams (800 calories)
Carbs= 357.5 grams (1,430 calories)
Fat= 70 grams (630 calories)

Chapter 6: Muscle Building Workout With Carb Cycling

Exercise is very important not only for your health but also for determining how your physique will look. If you want to build your best body possible, you must incorporate resistance training into your overall fitness plan. If you only use diet to lean down, something won't look quite right when you reach your goal bodyweight. Sure you'll have a low body fat percentage, but you'll end up looking flat, skinny and weak.

Resistance training is what stimulates your muscles to grow. However, your muscles don't actually grow when you're working out. During the workout, you're breaking down your muscle cells and telling your body to start the process of rebuilding them. It's during the recovery process, when you're getting plenty of rest and eating the right foods that your damaged muscles will start to grow back bigger and stronger.

Working out is what will get you a lean and defined look. Whether you're male or female, you don't have to overdue it and take on the look of an overly bulky bodybuilder. Additionally, weight training will also help prevent muscle loss (10). It basically comes down to the "use it or lose it" principle. If you restrict your calories and you aren't weight training, your body won't have any use for extra muscle, and it's more likely to use it for energy. Conversely, if you regularly lift weights, your body will keep that additional muscle mass because it knows that it'll need it sooner or later.

Workout to Build Muscle Mass Fast

The following training routine will consist of two different workouts—workout A and workout B. You'll alternate between workout A and workout B every time you go to the gym. You can workout 3 or 4 days per week; either way will get you results, so pick what works best for your schedule.

Here's how to set up your gym schedule if you want to workout three days per week:

Monday: Workout A
Tuesday: Rest Day
Wednesday: Workout B
Thursday: Rest Day
Friday: Workout A
Saturday: Rest Day
Sunday: Rest Day
Following Monday: Workout B

Or:

Monday: Rest Day
Tuesday: Workout A
Wednesday: Rest Day
Thursday: Workout B
Friday: Rest Day
Saturday: Workout A
Sunday: Rest Day
Following Tuesday: Workout B

And here's how to set up your gym schedule if you want to workout 4 days per week:

Monday: Workout A
Tuesday: Workout B

Wednesday: Rest Day
Thursday: Workout A
Friday: Workout B
Saturday: Rest Day
Sunday: Rest Day

Or:

Monday: Workout A
Tuesday: Workout B
Wednesday: Rest Day
Thursday: Workout A
Friday: Rest Day
Saturday: Workout B
Sunday: Rest Day

The second option will give your central nervous system an extra day of rest in-between your third and fourth workouts, which you may find beneficial. In the end though, pick whatever option works best for you and is the easiest for you to stick with.

Here are the actual workouts:

Workout A: Chest, Shoulders, and Triceps

- Incline Barbell or Dumbbell Bench Press: 3 sets of 6 reps 3 min rest btw (between) sets
- Standing Barbell Military Press: 3 sets of 6 reps 3 min rest btw sets
- Overhead Dumbbell Triceps Extension: 3 sets of 8 reps 90 sec rest btw sets
- Seated Dumbbell Lateral Raises: 3 sets of 10-12 reps 60 sec rest btw sets
- Face Pulls: 3 sets of 10-12 reps 60 sec rest btw sets
- Tricep Rope Pushdown: 3 sets of 12 reps 60 sec rest btw sets

Workout B: Back, Biceps, and Legs

- Weighted Pull-Ups (replace with lat pulldowns if you're unable to do pull-ups): 3 sets of 6 reps 3 min rest btw sets
- Barbell Back Squats: 3 sets of 8 reps 2 min rest btw sets
- Standing Dumbbell Curls: 3 sets of 8 reps 90 sec rest btw sets
- Bent Over Row: 3 sets of 8 reps 2 min rest btw sets
- Cross Body Hammer Curls: 3 sets of 10-12 reps 60 sec rest btw sets

Side Note: A set is a group of consecutive repetitions. A repetition is one complete motion of an exercise. And the rest period is how long of a break you'll take until you start the next set. For example, let's say you're completing 3 sets of 8 reps and resting 2 minutes in between sets for the barbell back squat exercise.

You'll squat down and stand back up, completing the motion of the exercise and one rep. You'll repeat that motion 7 more times for a total of 8 repetitions. That will complete the set and you will begin your rest period. Once your 2-minute rest period is up, you'll start the next set and perform another 8 repetitions.

That will complete set number 2, and you'll rest another 2 minutes. Once that time period is up, you'll complete the final set of 8 repetitions, and then you'll move onto the next exercise.

One of the reasons why I love this workout so much is because of the frequency. You'll be training each muscle group twice per week. This is important because muscle protein synthesis is increased in a muscle group for up to 48 hours after you train it (11). Muscle protein synthesis is the rate at which protein is being shuttled into and out of a particular muscle.

With a typical bro split, you'd be working out five days a week, and you'd only be training one muscle group per workout. The workout is typically set up like this:

Monday: Chest
Tuesday: Back
Wednesday: Legs
Thursday: Shoulders
Friday: Arms
Saturday: Rest Day
Sunday: Rest Day

The problem with this workout split is that you're only working out each muscle group one time per week! When you workout your chest on Monday, muscle protein synthesis will be increased in that area for 48 hours. Instead of training your chest again once that 48-hour period is up, you'll be waiting around for another four days before you workout chest again!

Who do you think would add more muscle to his chest over the course of a year?

Person A who works out his chest once a week for a total of 52 times a year.

Or:

Person B who works out his chest twice per week for a total of 104 times per year.

The answer is obvious. The reason why bro splits are so popular is because so many bodybuilders use them. However, there many be more to that than meets the eye and sometimes drugs could be a part of the equation.

Certain substances help them recover from their workouts faster than natural lifters like you and I. So while a bro split may be a good idea for a substance abusing bodybuilder, it has little use for us. Stick with the workout plan and get stronger with the given exercises. That's the best way to make gains quickly!

Chapter 7: What About Cardio?

Cardio is a very hot topic in the fitness community today. You hear about professional bodybuilders using it to lean down for competitions, but then you hear someone else bashing it for being too slow and boring.

So who's right in all of this? Hopefully, I can set you on the right path and give you a true understanding of what cardio is all about.

Is Cardio Even Necessary to Lose Weight?

The answer to the above question is definitely not! I can completely understand why many people think that they must do hours upon hours of cardio if they want to shred a few pounds. You hear all of the time about how fitness models and bodybuilders use cardio as a way to get absolutely shredded, so it's easy to believe it's required. However, cardio is not required at all to lose weight and get down to a low level of body fat.

What is required to lose weight and shred fat is eating less calories than your total daily energy expenditure as I mentioned earlier. It doesn't matter if you use exercise (i.e. cardio in this case) and/or diet to achieve that, both will get the job done. With that being said, it's much easier to control your total number of calories through your diet as opposed to exercising more. Think about it for a second.

What's easier- eating a slice of pizza and then doing 30 minutes of cardio to burn it off or not eating the slice of pizza in the first place? It's obvious; you shouldn't eat the pizza in the first place. Sure, you could try to burn off the extra calories every now and then, but it won't last for long. You're fighting an uphill battle because 30 minutes of your time isn't worth whatever it is that you want to eat so badly.

That's why you hear people say that you can't out exercise a bad diet. It's true, so focus more on your diet and the number of calories that you're eating instead of doing more cardio. Also, don't fret if you think this means that you'll have to give up your favorite foods to lose weight because it doesn't. You'll still get to enjoy your favorite foods *without* having to worry about weight gain or doing some extra cardio to make up for it.

How You Should Think About Cardio

From now on, I want you to think about cardio as a tool that can help you burn some extra calories instead of thinking of cardio as a requirement to do with carb cycling to lose weight. Cardio is one way to help get you below your total daily energy expenditure (TDEE), and you can use it when you feel that it's needed to get the job done.

As a single tool usually won't be enough to get the job done, cardio alone usually won't be enough to get you burning more calories than your TDEE. The main focus still needs to be on the carb cycling nutrition plan I outlined earlier. With this type of mindset, you'll only have to do cardio when you feel that it's necessary. It's important to note that moderate to high intensity cardio *isn't required* at all for carb cycling to work.

I believe that honing in on nutrition is the right way to go when trying to lose weight. This is because diet is the easiest and fastest way to control the total number of calories you're eating. However, once you have your diet in check, if you feel like adding in some extra exercise, then by all means do so.

Cardio can be a good way to speed up the fat loss process or at the very least give you some more leeway in your diet.

The Best Cardio Workout

With so many cardio workouts in existence today, which one is the best? Is it a slow steady state cardio? How about sprinting? Or maybe any type of cardio done on an empty stomach is the best?

The kind of cardio that you do doesn't matter much. This is because if the cardio workout doesn't put your total caloric intake below your TDEE (I know I keep bringing this up so it must be important, right?), then you won't be losing any weight.

So I would first and foremost recommend doing any type of cardio you enjoy whether that's walking, sprinting, jogging, swimming, kickboxing, etc. However, I will say the cardio workout I'll be providing you with here is the best way to go. It's a combination of high intensity interval training (HIIT) and slow steady state cardio. Research has shown higher intensity cardio results in more fat loss over time than lower intensity cardio (12) (13).

HIIT really is efficient—you're burning more calories in less time. HIIT's even cooler though when combined with slow steady state cardio. The reason why is because the HIIT will release free fatty acids into the bloodstream, and then the slow steady state cardio will burn off those free fatty acids.

Most people will do HIIT but won't follow it up with slow steady state cardio. This is a shame because all of those free fatty acids released into the bloodstream will get reabsorbed.

Here's how to do a combo cardio workout:

Note: This cardio workout can be done on any type of cardio machine (treadmill, elliptical, etc.), outside, on a track or wherever else you want. No matter where you are, the workout will be the same.

Combo Cardio Workout

#1: 10-15 minutes of HIIT on treadmill (or cardio machine of choice)

-Sprint for 30 seconds

-Walk for 1 minute (alternate between sprinting and walking for the full 10-15 min)

#2: Immediately followed by: 10-15 minutes of steady state cardio

-Walk on treadmill at 3.5 mph

Now the cool thing about HIIT is that you can adjust it to your current fitness level. For example if you can't sprint for 30 seconds, do a fast jog for 20 seconds (7.5 mph on a treadmill as an example) and then walk for 1 minute and 10 seconds.

You could even do 45 seconds of sprinting and 45 seconds of walking if you're in better shape. You can customize it to your needs, but you have the do the HIIT first followed by the slow steady state cardio.

I recommend that you do this 20-30 minute workout 2 times per week. I wouldn't advise that you do it anymore than 2 times per week because that's too much and it's not necessary beyond that point.

Final Cardio Considerations

Here's the deal:

You might not feel like doing HIIT sometimes. What do you do then? Luckily, you don't have to skip cardio altogether—there's an easier way and it's called walking. I recommend walking as much as you possibly can.

Walking is great because it can help to reduce stress (14) and speed up recovery from a hard workout. Walking also helps with lymphatic system recovery, and there's research showing how walking more (or moving more in general for that matter) can reduce your risk for developing heart disease (15).

Best of all, walking is an easy way to burn more calories. I used to think that walking was only for people who weren't in that good of shape, but boy was I wrong about that! Walking should be done by everyone, fit or unfit. The simple fact is that walking provides benefits that the higher intensity cardio can't.

I recommend going for walks around town or at the local park. Go outside and get some fresh air. Walking for 30 minutes 3 days a week would be enough to start providing you with some amazing benefits. You can still do the combination cardio workout twice per week in addition to the walking if you want to.

Chapter 8: 30 Low-Carb Recipes

Tilapia Parmesan

Ingredients:

- 2- 6 oz. tilapia fillets
- 2 tbsp. mayonnaise
- 2 tbsp. plain yogurt
- 1/4 cup parmesan cheese
- 3 sprigs fresh dill
- 1 tsp. garlic powder
- Black pepper to taste

Directions:

1. Put mayonnaise, yogurt and parmesan cheese in a small bowl and mix with a spoon.
2. Cover a cookie sheet with aluminum and spray with cooking spray.
3. Put oven to broil on high.
4. Put tilapia fillets roughly 2 inches apart on cookie sheet.
5. Divide cheese mixture evenly on each fillet.
6. Rub dill with fingers to separate roughly 1.5 sprigs worth of leaves over each fillet.
7. Sprinkle each fillet with half of garlic powder and season with salt and pepper.
8. Place cookie sheet into broiler.
9. Cook for 7-10 minutes, let cool and enjoy!

Number of servings: 2

Macros (per serving):

Calories: 275.2
Protein: 48.5 g
Carbs: 1.4 g
Fat: 8.5 g

*Recipe courtesy of LEXIBELLE715

Lime Chicken

Ingredients:

- 4 skinless and boneless chicken breasts
- 3 garlic cloves
- 1 cup salsa
- 1 1/2 worth lime juice
- 1/4 cup reduced fat ranch dressing
- 1 cup reduced fat cheddar cheese

Directions:

1. Spray skillet with cooking heat and place stove on medium heat.
2. Chop chicken breasts in half.
3. Sauté chicken for 3 minutes per side.
4. Add in garlic.
5. In a separate bowl, mix salsa, lime juice and ranch dressing.
6. Spread mixture onto the chicken.
7. Cook for another 5 minutes.
8. Add in the cheese and cook for another 5 minutes until chicken is no longer pink.

Number of servings: 8

Macros (per serving):

Calories: 208.9
Protein: 31.4 g
Carbs: 6.7 g
Fata: 6.2 g

*Recipe courtesy of VJB2601

Tuna Salad

Ingredients:

- 1 can albacore tuna
- 2/3 cup non-fat cottage cheese
- 4 tbsp. plain low-fat yogurt
- 1/4 small red onion, finely chopped
- 1 stalk celery, finely chopped
- 1 tsp. Dijon mustard
- Squirt of lemon juice
- A pinch of dill

Directions:

1. Mix all of the ingredients in a bowl and enjoy!

Number of servings: 2

Macros (per serving):

Calories: 190.3
Protein: 32.5 g
Carbs: 11.7 g
Fat: 2.2 g

*Recipe courtesy of GORGEOUS26

Parmesan Shrimp

Ingredients:

- 14 medium shrimp, peeled and deveined
- 1 tbsp. olive oil
- 1/2 clove garlic, minced
- 2 dashes of salt
- 1/4 tsp. Creole seasoning
- 2 dashes of ground pepper
- 1/8 cup Panko breadcrumbs
- 1 tbsp. shredded parmesan cheese

Directions:

1. Place shrimp, garlic, olive oil, salt, pepper and Creole seasoning into Ziploc bag.
2. Flip bag in multiple directions until shrimp is well coated.
3. Place in fridge for 1.5 hours.
4. Preheat oven to 475 degrees F.
5. Add bread crumbs and Parmesan to bag and turn until coated.
6. Spray a baking pan with butter and arrange shrimp on pan to where they don't touch.
7. Broil for roughly 10 minutes or until thoroughly cooked.
8. Add in the squeezed lemon and enjoy!

Number of servings: 2

Macros (per serving):

Calories: 137.6
Protein: 10.2 g
Carbs: 4.7 g
Fat: 8.6 g
*Recipe courtesy of PRAIRIEHARPY

Crustless Quiche

Ingredients:

- 1 cup non-fat cottage cheese
- 2 cups liquid egg whites
- 1/2 cup cooled broccoli
- 1/2 cup ham
- 1/2 cup low-fat Colby cheese
- Salt and pepper to taste

Directions:

1. Preheat oven to 375 degrees F.
2. Mix all of the ingredients into a large bowl.
3. Spray a pie dish with cooking spray.
4. Put mixture into pie dish.
5. Put dish into oven, bake for 45 minutes and enjoy!

Number of servings: 6

Macros (per serving):

Calories: 106.8
Protein: 18.7 g
Carbs: 4.5 g
Fat: 1.4 g

*Recipe courtesy of CHESSMANS2000

Chicken Burgers

Ingredients:

- 1 lb. ground chicken
- 6 oz. crumbled feta
- 1 tbsp. ground oregano
- 1/4 tsp. salt
- 1/4 tsp. garlic powder

Directions:

1. Preheat broiler or grill.
2. Mix all of the ingredients together and form into 4 separate patties.
3. Grill or broil patties until internal temperature of burgers reaches 165 degrees F (approximately 8 minutes per side).
4. Serve and enjoy!

Number of servings: 4

Macros (per serving):

Calories: 285.6
Protein: 26.8 g
Carbs: 3.3 g
Fat: 19.8 g

*Recipe courtesy of PRAIRIEHARPY

Salmon Cakes

Ingredients:

- 1 can wild Alaskan Pink Salmon
- 1 cup raw onion
- 1 tsp. black pepper
- 1 tsp. garlic powder
- 1 large egg
- salt to taste

Directions:

1. Mix all of the ingredients together.
2. For mixture into 4 separate patties.
3. Fry patties similar to the way you would a burger until thoroughly cooked.

Number of servings: 4

Macros (per serving):

Calories: 195.0
Protein: 23.2 g
Carbs: 4.5 g
Fat: 10.1 g

*Recipe courtesy of MYTHINKER

Teriyaki Meatballs

Ingredients:

- 1 lb. lean ground beef
- 1/2 cup chopped green onions
- 1/3 cup teriyaki sauce
- 3 tsp. chopped ginger root

Directions:

1. Preheat oven to 350 degrees F.
2. Mix all of the ingredients together in a separate bowl.
3. Form 8- 2 oz. balls with the mixture.
4. Place the balls into a dish and bake for 25-30 minutes.

Number of servings: 8

Macros (per serving):

Calories: 101.1
Protein: 13.1 g
Carbs: 3.8 g
Fat: 3.5 g

*Recipe courtesy of PRAIRIEHARPY

Chicken Alfredo Bake

Ingredients:

- 3 boneless skinless chicken breasts
- 1 tbsp. cooking oil
- Montreal seasoning
- 1 cup cubed yellow squash
- 1 medium diced sweet onion
- 1 cup cauliflower
- salt and pepper to taste
- 1 jar Alfredo sauce
- 1/4 cup grated parmesan cheese
- 1/8 cup bread crumbs

Directions:

1. Preheat oven to 350 degrees F.
2. Spray 13x9 pan with cooking spray.
3. Sprinkle Montreal seasoning over chicken breasts and cook in skillet until there's no pink.
4. Put cauliflower in dish, add 2 tbsp. water, cover with plastic wrap and cook in microwave for 4 minutes.
5. Sauté cooking oil and onions until clear. Add in squash and sauté until soft.
6. Cut chicken into cubes and add to casserole dish with vegetable. Pour Alfredo sauce over the top of dish.
7. Top with cheese and bread crumbs and bake for 20 minutes, and then boil for 10 until top of dish is brown.

Number of servings: 8

Macros (per serving):

Calories: 240.1
Protein: 26.9 g
Carbs: 6.9 g

Fat: 12.0 g

*Recipe courtesy of PRAIRIEHARPY

Lettuce Wraps

Ingredients:

- 3.5 oz. lean ground beef
- 1 tbsp. finely minced onion
- 1 clove crushed minced garlic
- Dash garlic powder
- Dash dried oregano
- Chopped cilantro to taste
- Cayenne pepper to taste
- Salt and pepper to taste
- Lettuce leaves

Directions:

1. Brown ground beef until thoroughly cooked.
2. Add onion, garlic, spices, and a little water and simmer for 7-10 minutes.
3. Add salt to taste.
4. Add mixture onto lettuce, wrap it up, and enjoy!

Number of servings: 1

Macros (per serving):

Calories: 143.5
Protein: 21.7 g
Carbs: 4.2 g
Fat: 1.4 g

*Recipe courtesy of LIZZY63

Scrambled Eggs

Ingredients:

- 1/4 cup green bell pepper, finely chopped
- 1 tbsp. onion, finely chopped
- 2 large eggs
- 1/4 cup low-fat cottage cheese
- 2 tbsp. low-fat cheddar cheese
- 2 tbsp. salsa

Directions:

1. Beat eggs and cottage cheese together.
2. Spray nonstick skillet with cooking spray.
3. Cook peppers and onions on medium heat until tender, roughly 2 minutes.
4. Add egg mixture and cheddar cheese.
5. Reduce heat to medium. Cook until set, stirring as needed.
6. Put the salsa on top and enjoy!

Number of servings: 1

Macros (per serving):

Calories: 274.8
Protein: 24.3 g
Carbs: 7.9 g
Fat: 14.5 g

*Recipe courtesy of SOOKIE

Pork Chops for Crockpot

Ingredients:

- 10 pork chops
- 1 can low fat chicken cream soup
- 1/2 cup ketchup

Directions:

1. Put the pork chops into the crockpot.
2. Add in the soup and ketchup.
3. Cover the crockpot and cook on low for 8-9 hours.
4. Serve and enjoy!

Number of servings: 10

Macros (per serving):

Calories: 239.7
Protein: 21.8 g
Carbs: 8.2 g
Fat: 12.1 g

*Recipe courtesy of LASTX70

Country Style Crockpot Pork Ribs

Ingredients:

- 1/4 tsp. ground allspice
- 1/4 tsp. ground cinnamon
- 2 pounds country-style pork ribs
- 1/4 cup diced onion
- 1/2 tsp. garlic powder
- 1 tbsp. sugar-free maple-flavored syrup
- 1 dash black pepper
- 1/4 tsp. ground ginger
- 1 tbsp. low-sodium soy sauce

Directions:

1. Mix all of the ingredients into a bowl minus the ribs.
2. Pour mixture over ribs.
3. Put ribs in crockpot and cook for 8-9 hours on low.
4. Cover with foil and bake for 60-90 minutes if baking in oven.

Number of servings: 4

Macros (per serving):

Calories: 188.4
Protein: 22.3 g
Carbs: 2.3 g
Fat: 9.4 g

*Recipe courtesy of LANDMOM

Cottage Cheese Breakfast

Ingredients:

- 1 cup 1% cottage cheese
- 1 tsp. ground cinnamon
- 1 packet Splenda
- 1/4 cup chopped almonds

Directions:

1. Put the cottage cheese, cinnamon, and Splenda in a bowl and mix well.
2. Sprinkle the chopped almonds on top and enjoy!

Number of servings: 1

Macros (per serving):

Calories: 249.8
Protein: 30.8 g
Carbs: 14.9 g
Fat: 8.6 g

*Recipe courtesy of NURSEHOPE

Tuna Burgers

Ingredients:

- 2 cups tuna
- 1/3 cup tomato sauce
- 1/4 cup finely chopped dill pickle onions
- 2 egg whites
- 1/4 cup wholegrain flour
- 1/4 tsp. black pepper
- 1/2 tsp. garlic powder
- 1/2 tsp. onion powder

Directions:

1. Put all of the ingredients in a bowl and thoroughly mix together.
2. Form mixture into 4 separate patties.
3. Spray skillet with cooking spray and cook on medium-high heat until thoroughly cooked on each side.
4. Serve and enjoy!

Number of servings: 4

Macros (per serving):

Calories: 140.5
Protein: 23.7 g
Carbs: 8.5 g
Fat: 1.3 g

*Recipe courtesy of FLOWERDALEJEWEL

Cheddar Bread

Ingredients:

- 1 large egg
- 2 tsp. flax seed meal
- 1/2 tbsp. baking powder
- 1 packet Splenda
- 1/4 cup shredded cheddar cheese
- 1 tsp. melted butter

Directions:

1. Melt butter in flat bowl or 15 oz. oval ramekin.
2. Add in the egg, flax meal, baking powder, Splenda, cheddar cheese and mix well.
3. Put in the microwave for 1 minute.
4. Flip over and cook for another 10 seconds until cooked throughout.
5. Cut in half, serve with favorite sandwich fillings and enjoy!

Number of servings: 1

Macros (per serving):

Calories: 289.2
Protein: 16.4 g
Carbs: 5.4 g
Fat: 22.5 g

*Recipe courtesy of XANADUREALM

Scampi Shrimp

Ingredients:

- 1 tbsp. canola oil
- 3/4 lb. uncooked peeled and deveined shrimp
- 1 med diced green onion
- 1/4 tsp. garlic powder
- 1/2 tsp. basil
- 3/4 tsp. parsley
- 1 tbsp. lemon juice
- 3 tbsp. parmesan cheese

Directions:

1. Heat oil over medium heat in 10" skillet.
2. Add shrimp and remaining ingredients to skillet.
3. Cook for 5-7 minutes.
4. Remove skillet from heat and sprinkle with Parmesan cheese.
5. Serve and enjoy!

Number of servings: 4

Macros (per serving):

Calories: 143.5
Protein: 19.0 g
Carbs: 2.1 g
Fat: 6.1 g

*Recipe courtesy of JOELSANGEL

No-Carb Cajun Tilapia

Ingredients:

- 4 oz. tilapia filet
- 1 tsp. extra virgin olive oil
- 1/2 tbsp. unsalted butter
- Favorite Cajun spice of your choosing to taste

Directions:

1. Melt butter and olive oil in a skillet.
2. Cover fish with Cajun spice.
3. Cook fish fillet in butter and oil for 3-5 minutes per side until thoroughly cooked.
4. Serve and enjoy!

Number of servings: 1

Macros (per serving):

Calories: 143.9
Protein: 21.0 g
Carbs: 0.0 g
Fat: 6.3 g

*Recipe courtesy of THEBERT99

Regular Chicken Salad

Ingredients:

- 1 1/2 cups cooked and chopped chicken
- 1 1/2 cups chopped celery
- 3 tbsp. light mayonnaise
- 1 tsp. mustard
- Salt and pepper to taste

Directions:

1. Put all of the ingredients together in a bowl and thoroughly mix together.

Number of servings: 1

Macros (per serving):

Calories: 173.8
Protein: 24.2 g
Carbs: 3.5 g
Fat: 6.3 g

*Recipe courtesy of JTDALZELL

Chocolate Cheesecake

Ingredients:

For Sauce:
- 2 tbsp. butter
- 4 tbsp. cocoa
- 3 tbsp. Splenda

For Cake:
- 16 oz. cream cheese
- 1 pkg. of sugar free instant chocolate pudding mix
- 1/2 cup of heavy cream
- 1/2 cup of Splenda
- 1 tsp. vanilla extract
- 2 eggs

Directions:

For Sauce:

1. Melt together butter, cocoa and Splenda (3 tbsp. worth) on stovetop or in microwave.

For Cake:

1. Preheat oven to 350 degrees F.
2. Mix together cream cheese, Splenda, vanilla and eggs.
3. Mix heavy cream and pudding together in separate bowl from other mixture.
4. Combine both mixtures toughly in blender.
5. Spray a pie plate with cooking spray.
6. Put cheesecake mixture in pan and place in oven for around 40 minutes.
7. Remove and drizzle sauce on top. Refrigerate, serve cold and enjoy!

Number of servings: 12

Macros (per serving):

Calories: 207.7
Protein: 4.8 g
Carbs: 5.4 g
Fat: 20.0 g

*Recipe courtesy of JNORMAN1969

Cauliflower Faux Mashed Potatoes

Ingredients:

- 1 head raw cauliflower (5-6 in. in diameter)
- 1/4 cup sour cream
- 2 tbsp. salted butter

Directions:

1. Steam cauliflower until soft.
2. Put cooked cauliflower in a pot and heat to get rid of the excess moisture.
3. Puree cauliflower in food processor.
4. Add butter and sour cream and enjoy!

Number of servings: 4

Macros (per serving):

Calories: 117.6
Protein: 3.4 g
Carbs: 8.1 g
Fat: 9.1 g

*Recipe courtesy of ARTEMISINKED

Chicken Noodle Soup

Ingredients:

- 1 package fettuccini noodles
- 1 cup chopped onion
- 1 cup chopped cabbage
- 1 cup spinach
- 1 cup chopped carrots
- 1 clove garlic
- 1 tsp. ginger
- 1 tsp. red pepper flakes
- 8 oz. chicken
- 4 cups broth
- 1 tbsp. soy sauce

Directions:

1. Rinse fettuccini noodles under warm water for 30 seconds, drain, and let air dry while preparing other ingredients.
2. Boil the 4 cups of broth.
3. Add all of the ingredients to the broth (noodles included) and cook for 6-7 minutes until vegetables become tender.

Number of servings: 4

Macros (per serving):

Calories: 174.5
Protein: 18.8 g
Carbs: 11.8 g
Fat: 6.1 g

*Recipe courtesy of CLYNNTHOMAS

Beef and Turkey Meatloaf

Ingredients:

- 3 1/2 lbs. ground turkey
- 3 1/2 lbs. ground beef
- 1 cup chopped onion
- 1 cup shredded carrots
- 1 sleeve saltine crackers
- 1/2 cup non-fat milk
- 4 large eggs
- 1 tbsp. salt
- 1 tbsp. pepper
- 2 tbsp. Worcestershire sauce
- 6 chopped cloves of garlic

Directions:

1. Preheat oven to 350 degrees F.
2. In a large bowl, crumble up the crackers and soak them in the milk for 15 minutes.
3. Chop the vegetables and add remaining ingredients to the cracker bowl.
4. Mix all of the ingredients in the bowl together until combined.
5. Form the combined mixture into a rectangle load in a 13x9 baking dish.
6. Bake for 80-90 minutes or until internal temp. reaches 160 degrees.
7. Cool for 10 minutes, serve, and enjoy!

Number of servings: 12

Macros (per serving):

Calories: 467.1
Protein: 21.7 g
Carbs: 8.5 g

Fat: 31.7 g

*Recipe courtesy of CLYNNTHOMAS

Chicken Enchiladas

Ingredients:

- 2 skinless chicken breasts
- 1 can cream chicken soup
- 1 can cream mushroom soup
- 1/4 cup diced green chilies
- 1 cup salsa verde
- 1/4 cup chopped tomatoes
- 8 whole-wheat tortillas
- 2 cups Colby jack cheese

Directions:

1. Preheat oven to 350 degrees F.
2. Boil the chicken breast and shred when cooled.
3. Mix cream chicken and cream mushroom soups, cheese, chilies, salsa verde and tomatoes together in large bowl.
4. Remove half of the mixture from the bowl and set aside for later use.
5. Add shredded chicken remaining mixture in bowl.
6. Lay a tortilla flat and fill with about 3 tsp. of the chicken, then repeat this process for the remaining tortillas.
7. Pour the rest of the mixture you set aside earlier over the top of the enchiladas and bake for 45 minutes.
8. Cool for 15 minutes and enjoy!

Number of servings: 8

Macros (per serving):

Calories: 155.4
Protein: 13.9 g

Carbs: 4.2 g
Fat: 7.3 g

*Recipe courtesy of KFOX05

Protein Shake

Ingredients:

- 1 scoop (roughly 33 grams) vanilla cream whey protein powder
- 8 oz. unsweetened almond breeze vanilla almond milk
- 6 ice cubes
- 1 tsp. of vanilla extract

Directions:

1. Put all of the ingredients together in a blender and blend until smooth.

Number of servings: 1

Macros (per serving):

Calories: 170.0
Protein: 24.0 g
Carbs: 8.0 g
Fat: 4.5 g

*Recipe courtesy of LISAM67

Veggie Bacon Cheese Omlet

Ingredients:

- 1/4 cup liquid egg whites
- 1/4 cup raw onions
- 1/4 cup chopped green peppers
- 1/4 cup chopped tomatoes
- 1/4 cup reduced fat feta cheese
- 1/4 serving pre-cooked bacon

Directions:

1. Spray skillet with cooking spray and place on medium heat.
2. Add in peppers and onions and sauté for a bit until crisp.
3. Tear apart the bacon and add to skillet.
4. Add in the egg mixture and mix together with other ingredients.
5. Put the tomatoes and feta cheese on top and continue stirring until done.

Number of servings: 1

Macros (per serving):

Calories: 170.3
Protein: 20.3 g
Carbs: 9.6 g
Fat: 4.9 g

*Recipe courtesy of NATNEAGLE

Pumpkin Spice Frappuccino

Ingredients:

- 3/4 tsp. pumpkin spice
- 1-2 tsp. instant coffee
- 3 tbsp. canned pumpkin
- 1 tsp. stevia
- 2 tsp. sugar twin
- 3 tbsp. French vanilla coffee creamer
- 1 cup unsweetened coconut milk
- 6 ice cubes

Directions:

1. Put all of the ingredients in a blender and blend until mixture is smooth.

Number of servings: 2

Macros (per serving):

Calories: 66.3
Protein: 0.6 g
Carbs: 3.3 g
Fat: 4.7 g

*Recipe courtesy of MISTYRIOS

Taco Salad

Ingredients:

- 1 lb. extra lean ground beef
- 1 pkg. old El Paso taco seasoning
- 3/4 cup water
- 2 tbsp. olive oil
- 4 cups shredded romaine lettuce
- 1/2 cup chopped tomatoes
- 8 tbsp. fat free sour cream
- 1 cup shredded cheddar cheese

Directions:

1. Chop lettuce and set aside with tomatoes, cheese and sour cream.
2. Brown the beef with olive oil in skillet until thoroughly cooked.
3. Add in the taco seasoning and water to the skillet.
4. Simmer until water is reduced and remove from heat when done.
5. In 4 bowls, put one cup of lettuce in each bowl.
6. Add ¼ cup chopped tomatoes, beef, and cheese to each bowl.
7. Then add two tbsp. of sour cream to each bowl, serve and enjoy!

Number of servings: 4

Macros (per serving):

Calories: 489.0
Protein: 31.0 g
Carbs: 9.6 g
Fat: 36.1 g

*Recipe courtesy of TOASTERGIRL

Snicker doodle Cookies

Ingredients:

- 1/2 cup butter
- 1 1/2 cup almond flour
- 1 cup Splenda
- 1 egg
- 1/2 tsp. vanilla
- 1/4 tsp. baking soda
- 1/4 tsp. cream of tartar
- 2 tbs. Splenda
- 1 tsp. cinnamon

Directions:

1. Mix together all of the ingredients minus the cinnamon and Splenda.
2. Cover the bowl and refrigerate for 1 hour.
3. In a separate bowl, mix together the cinnamon and Splenda.
4. Roll dough in small balls throughout Splenda and cinnamon mixture.
5. Place dough balls on mixture and bake in oven at 350 degrees F for 15 minutes.
6. Remove and cool for 10 minutes and enjoy!

Number of servings: 20

Macros (per serving):

Calories: 99.1
Protein: 2.5 g
Carbs: 4.4 g
Fat: 9.4 g

*Recipe courtesy of SHELLSLYN

Chile Casserole

Ingredients:

- 2- 7 oz. cans of green chilies
- 8 oz. shredded pepper-jack cheese
- 3 eggs
- 3/4 cup heavy cream
- 1/2 tsp. salt
- 4 oz. shredded cheddar cheese

Directions:

1. Grease an 8x8-baking pan and preheat oven to 350 degrees F.
2. Slice each chili along the long side and open to where it lays flat.
3. Arrange half of the chilies on one side of the pan, skin side down in a single layer.
4. Top the chilies with pepper-jack cheese.
5. Put the remaining chilies on top of the cheese, skin side up.
6. Beat the eggs, cream, and salt well, and then pour over the chilies.
7. Top with cheddar cheese and bake in oven for 35 minutes or until golden brown.
8. Let it cool off for 12 minutes, serve and enjoy!

Number of servings: 9

Macros (per serving):

Calories: 211.0
Protein: 10.9 g
Carbs: 1.4 g
Fat: 17.6 g

*Recipe courtesy of THELMAGADDIS

Chapter 9: 15 High-Carb Recipes

Meat and Potatoes Dinner

Ingredients:

- 1 large potato
- 4 baby carrots
- 1/4 cup of onion
- 3 mushrooms
- Pat of butter
- 3 oz. extra lean ground beef
- Salt and pepper to taste

Directions:

1. Preheat oven to 450 degrees F.
2. Put a large piece of foil over a cookie sheet, spread butter over it, chop all of the vegetables (including potato), and put them on the sheet.
3. Put the hamburger chunks over the vegetables.
4. Roll the foil so the vegetables and beef stay inside.
5. Place the sheet in the oven and bake for 30 minutes.
6. Remove, let it cool and enjoy!

Number of servings: 1

Macros (per serving):

Calories: 564.1
Protein: 26.3 g
Carbs: 73.5 g

Fat: 19.4 g

*Recipe courtesy of RDEFASSI

Chocolate Chip Cookies

Ingredients:

- 2 1/2 cups white flour
- 3/4 cup granulated sugar
- 3 cups old fashioned Quaker oats
- 2 cups chopped walnuts
- 2 cups chocolate chips
- 2 sticks margarine butter
- 1 tsp. salt
- 1 tsp. baking soda
- 1 cup whey protein powder
- 1 tsp. vanilla flavoring
- 3 eggs

Directions:

1. Preheat oven to 350 degrees F
2. Cream the sugars and margarine butter.
3. Add in vanilla and eggs and beat until smooth.
4. Add in protein powder then salt, baking powder, and flour and mix until smooth.
5. Add in the chocolate chips, oatmeal and walnuts and stir until smooth.
6. Use a ¼ measuring cup to portion the dough and make each cookie roughly 3" in diameter and ½" high.
7. Bake for around 10 minutes until golden brown.
8. Let them sit and cool and enjoy!

Number of servings: 48

Macros (per serving):

Calories: 168.6
Protein: 6.5 g
Carbs: 18.8 g

Fat: 8.7 g

*Recipe courtesy of STIURF

Dinner Rolls

Ingredients:

- 1/4 cup honey
- 1 cup warm water
- 1 envelope yeast
- 1/3 cup non-fat dry milk
- 1/3 cup unsalted melted butter
- 2 eggs
- 1 tsp. salt
- 4 1/2 cups flour

Directions:

1. Dissolve honey and yeast in warm water and let it stand until foamy.
2. Add in the milk powder, butter, eggs and salt then stir.
3. Gradually add in the flour and knead for 8 minutes.
4. Let the dough rise until doubled in height, press them down again and let them rise for 30 minutes before putting them in the oven.
5. Form into 30 round rolls and place them on the baking sheet.
6. Bake in the oven at 375 degrees F for 15 minutes.
7. Let cool for 10 minutes, serve and enjoy!

Number of servings: 30

Macros (per serving):

Calories: 80.5
Protein: 2.3 g
Carbs: 14.8 g
Fat: 1.2 g

*Recipe courtesy of BKMNURSING

Ham and Green Bean Dinner

Ingredients:

- 2 lbs. quarter ham roast
- 6 medium sized potatoes
- 12 oz. can green beans
- 1 cup ginger ale

Directions:

1. Preheat oven to 450 degrees F.
2. Put ham roast on a baking pan and add one cup of ginger ale.
3. Place potatoes on separate pan and bake them at the same time as the ham roast.
4. Bake for about 35 minutes or until thoroughly cooked.
5. Boil the green beans while the ham roast and potatoes are baking on medium heat.
6. Serve and enjoy!

Number of servings: 6

Macros (per serving):

Calories: 190.7
Protein: 8.4 g
Carbs: 36.4 g
Fat: 1.5 g

*Recipe courtesy of NICOLE_SANTILLO

Salmon and Rice Dinner

Ingredients:

- 4 oz. wild salmon
- 1/2 cup whole grain brown rice
- 1 cup chopped broccoli
- 2 tsp. Parmesan grated cheese
- Sea salt to taste
- Garlic powder to taste
- Onion powder to taste
- Parsley to taste

Directions:

1. Preheat oven to broil.
2. Place salmon on non-stick pan with the scales facing down.
3. Season salmon with the sea salt, parsley, onion powder and garlic powder.
4. Bake the salmon for about 15 minutes.
5. While the salmon is baking, make the rice according to pkg. directions.
6. Then steam the broccoli until thoroughly heated.
7. When done, put the rice in a bowl and grate with Parmesan cheese.
8. Put rice on top of broccoli, remove the salmon and place on rice and enjoy!

Number of servings: 1

Macros (per serving):

Calories: 340.0
Protein: 29.0 g
Carbs: 32.0 g
Fat: 8.0 g
*Recipe courtesy of FAYETTESIDRA

Beef Hamburger

Ingredients:

- 6 oz. lean ground beef
- 1 hamburger bun
- 1 tbsp. light mayonnaise
- 1 tbsp. ketchup
- 1 tbsp. yellow mustard
- Toppings of your choosing

Directions:

1. Cook the ground beef on a skillet over medium heat until thoroughly cooked and there's no pink.
2. Toast the bun in a toaster.
3. Put 1 tbsp. of mayo on the bottom half of the bun.
4. Put the patty on the bottom half of the bun.
5. Add in the ketchup and mustard.
6. Put any additional toppings on the burger that you like.
7. Place the top bun on and enjoy!

Number of servings: 1

Macros (per serving):

Calories: 458.4
Protein: 38.9 g
Carbs: 26.9 g
Fat: 22.0 g

*Recipe courtesy of WHITEBOY23

Sausage and Black Beans

Ingredients:

- 1 tbsp. flour
- 2- 15 oz. cans black beans
- 2- 10 oz. packages frozen kernel corn
- 16 oz. jar chunky salsa
- 1 lb. smoked sliced sausage
- 1 cup Colby jack cheese

Directions:

1. Preheat oven to 450 degrees F.
2. In a large bowl, mix together the flour, beans, corn, salsa and sliced sausage.
3. Put the mixed ingredients in a large, extra heavy-duty foil bag in a 1-inch deep pan, arranged in an even layer.
4. Double fold the bag and seal it
5. Bake in the oven for 50-60 minutes.
6. Once done, hold the bag with mitts and cut it open with a knife.
7. Cautiously, fold back the top of the bag so the steam can escape.
8. Sprinkle with cheese, serve, and enjoy!

Number of servings: 5

Macros (per serving):

Calories: 546.4
Protein: 33.3 g
Carbs: 69.8 g
Fat: 14.9 g

*Recipe courtesy of CASSIDYR

Crockpot Turkey Dinner

Ingredients:

- 3/4 lb. turkey breast
- 1 can Campbell's cream of chicken soup
- 1/2 pkg. dry French onion soup mix
- 2 1/4 cup water
- 1 cup dry pearled barley
- 3 cups frozen green beans

Directions:

1. Put the turkey, soup mixes and 3/4 cup of water into the crockpot and cook on low for 6 hours.
2. After 6 hours have passed, add in the barley, remaining water and green beans, and continue cooking in the crockpot for an additional hour.
3. Serve and enjoy!

Number of servings: 6

Macros (per serving):

Calories: 328.0
Protein: 37.1 g
Carbs: 38.2 g
Fat: 2.5 g

*Recipe courtesy of GVMEMOMENT

Beef Spaghetti

Ingredients:

- 1 lb. lean ground beef
- 1/2 chopped onion
- 1/2 chopped green pepper
- 10 oz. drained canned mushrooms
- 28 oz. can diced tomatoes
- 8 oz. spaghetti, broken into 1-inch pieces
- 1 cup water
- 1 1/2 tsp. Italian seasoning
- Salt and pepper to taste

Directions:

1. In a large saucepan, brown the beef and onions over medium heat until the meat is no longer pink.
2. Throw in the green pepper and mushrooms and cook for a few more minutes.
3. Then add in the diced tomatoes, spaghetti and water and stir the mixture.
4. Add in the spices.
5. Cook and cover for 15 minutes, stirring occasionally or finish when spaghetti is tender.

Number of servings: 6

Macros (per serving):

Calories: 388.5
Protein: 21.1 g
Carbs: 38.7 g
Fat: 16.5 g

*Recipe courtesy of RAGGEDY_ANN

Calamari Salad

Ingredients:

For Salad:
- 3 cups tossed salad
- 1 large hardboiled egg, sliced in half
- 1/2 avocado
- 4 tbsp. shredded cheddar cheese
- 1 cubic inch crumbled feta cheese
- 8 pieces sun dried tomato

For Salad Garnish and Dressing:
- 2 lemon wedges
- 2 tsp. of olive oil
- Salt and pepper to taste

For Squid:
- 200 grams raw squid
- Salt and black pepper to taste
- 2 tsp. olive oil

Directions:

1. Slice the squid into rings, place in a bowl and drizzle with 2 tsp. of olive oil.
2. Add in salt and pepper, toss around to coat and let sit for 5 minutes.
3. Divide salad ingredients on two plates, using any other veggies you like.
4. Heat a skillet on medium heat and dump squid mixture onto skillet, sautéing for 7-10 minutes.
5. Divide squid on two plates and drizzle one tsp. of olive on each plate. Add salt and pepper and a lemon wedge to each and enjoy!

Number of servings: 2

Macros (per serving):

Calories: 418.5
Protein: 28.1 g
Carbs: 19.6 g
Fat: 26.6 g

*Recipe courtesy of KALEXIAS

Macaroni and Cheese Tuna Casserole

Ingredients:

- 1 box Kraft Mac N Cheese
- 1/4 cup skim milk
- 3 tsp. margarine
- 1 can tuna

Directions:

1. Boil the mac n cheese for about 8 minutes according to the box's instructions.
2. Drain the pasta.
3. Add in 1/4 cup of skim milk and stir.
4. Add in 3 tsp. of margarine and stir.
5. Add in the packet of cheese that comes with the macaroni and mix it in well.
6. Flake the tuna in the can with a fork and then add it to the macaroni and stir well.

Number of servings: 4

Macros (per serving):

Calories: 333.2
Protein: 27.6 g
Carbs: 39.8 g
Fat: 5.6 g

*Recipe courtesy of SUMMERRAINCITY

Tortellini & Bacon Dinner

Ingredients:

- 2 cups frozen tortellini
- 4 slices diced bacon
- 3 tbsp. chopped parsley
- 1 small yellow onion
- 1/2 cup Parmesan cheese
- Salt and pepper to taste

Directions:

1. Cook the frozen tortellini according to package directions and set to the side.
2. Cook the bacon until the pieces are golden brown.
3. Place the bacon bits on a paper towel to help drain the excess fat.
4. Cook the chopped onions on the same skillet used to cook the bacon until caramelized.
5. Put the bacon bits, tortellini and parsley back in and cook for another 3 minutes.
6. Next add in the Parmesan cheese and cook until it melts.
7. Serve and enjoy!

Number of servings: 4

Macros (per serving):

Calories: 230.3
Protein: 11.4 g
Carbs: 27.2 g
Fat: 8.4 g

*Recipe courtesy of MYLEHIA

Turkey Tenderloin Stir Fry

Ingredients:

- 8 oz. diced turkey cutlets
- 2 cups chopped Swiss chard
- 3 cloves garlic
- 1 medium onion
- 1 cup chopped green bell peppers
- 1 cup chopped mushrooms
- 1/2 cup chopped water chestnuts
- 1 cup chopped broccoli
- 3 tbsp. soy sauce
- 1/2 cup chicken broth
- 6 tsp. granulated sugar
- 2 tbsp. cornstarch
- 1 tbsp. peanut oil
- 3 tsp. ginger root

Directions:

1. Heat oil in pan and cook peppers and onions until lightly cooked.
2. Throw in the garlic and cook for a few additional minutes.
3. Cook the turkey tenderloins until golden brown.
4. Throw in the vegetables and sauté until lightly cooked.
5. Mix together the soy sauce, cornstarch, and chicken broth. Add this mixture to the stir-fry and cook until it slightly thickens.

Number of servings: 2

Macros (per serving):

Calories: 396.1
Protein: 34.5 g
Carbs: 51.1 g

Fat: 8.1 g

*Recipe courtesy of CSPEAKE

Venison Pot Roast

Ingredients:

- 2 1/2 lbs. venison
- 1/2 tsp. black pepper
- 1/4 tsp. salt
- 2 sliced large onions
- 1 3/4 cup water
- 1 packet onion soup mix
- 1 1/2 tbsp. balsamic vinegar
- 1 tsp. dried thyme
- 8 medium red potatoes
- 2 cups baby carrots

Directions:

1. Preheat oven to 350 degrees F.
2. Coat a pot with cooking spray and heat over medium heat.
3. Put the roast in the pan and sprinkle with salt and pepper and then place the onions around the roast.
4. Cook the roast and onions for roughly 8 minutes until they brown.
5. Add water into the pot and then stir in the soup mix, vinegar, and thyme and bring to a boil.
6. Move the roast and onions to a 9x13 pan and bake in the oven for 1 hour.
7. Put the potatoes and carrots around the roast, then cover and bake for another 2 hours until the vegetables are tender.
8. Finally, put the roast on a cutting board and slice it against the grain, then serve and enjoy!

Number of servings: 10

Macros (per serving):

Calories: 292.9
Protein: 29.4 g
Carbs: 33.0 g
Fat: 2.3 g

*Recipe courtesy of CASCHWARTZ620

Italian Sausage and Rice

Ingredients:

- 1- 6 oz. pkg. chicken rice
- 1 lb. bulk Italian sausage
- 1 cup chopped onion
- 1 clove minced garlic
- 1 cup water
- 1- 16 oz. can peeled whole tomatoes
- 1 tsp. basil leaves
- 2 cups chopped broccoli
- 1 cup grated mozzarella cheese
- 2 tbsp. chopped parsley

Directions:

1. Brown the sausage, onion and garlic in a large skillet.
2. Add in the water, tomatoes and basil, and bring to a boil.
3. Add in the rice, reduce the heat and simmer for 15 minutes.
4. Add the broccoli and cook for another 7-10 minutes until liquid is absorbed.
5. Remove the skillet from heat, and then sprinkle with mozzarella cheese and parsley.
6. Cover and let it sit for 5 minutes, and then serve and enjoy!

Number of servings: 48

Macros (per serving):

Calories: 599.8
Protein: 29.6 g
Carbs: 38.9 g
Fat: 36.3 g
*Recipe courtesy of JAMIECEE

Chapter 10: How to Track Your Calories and Macros

Tracking your calories and macros is imperative if you want to see success with carb cycling. This is going to be the most tedious part of the process, but it has to be done. If you don't measure how many carbs and calories you're consuming, you won't have a clue if you're actually eating low carbs on the days you're supposed to. Fortunately, there are some ways to make tracking your calories and macros easier.

The simplest and easiest way to track your calories and macronutrients is to go to the App Store or Google Play Store, type in macro tracker and download one of the many apps available. Any of the worthwhile apps will cost you a few dollars, but it'll pay for itself over and over again considering all of the time it'll save you. Once you download an app, all you have to do is type in the foods you eat. The app will then tell you how many calories the food has as well as its protein, carb and fat contents. The majority of the apps will even contain a handy bar code scanner, which will allow you to instantly scan and store calories and macros from whatever you eat.

The other thing that makes an app so useful is the fact that it's on your phone, which will be with you wherever you go. If you decide to go out to eat dinner, for example, you'll still be able to track your calories right then and there. Don't wait and tell yourself that you'll remember everything you ate. Track it as soon as possible for the best results!

Another item you'll want to invest in is a food scale. These are pretty cheap, and you can buy one on Amazon for about $11. A food scale will tell you the amount of grams or ounces that are in the foods you're eating. You can then use the formulas from the earlier chapters to calculate the number of calories in the food items. This will be very useful to be able to measure out serving sizes as closely as possible. For example, if a nutritional label says that one serving of steak is 32 grams, you'll have no way of knowing if you're actually eating 32 grams unless you measure it.

If you decide not to use your phone to track your macros then you'll have to measure everything by hand using a notebook, which can be extremely inconvenient. Tracking your calories in this manner will become a pain-in-the-neck rather quickly, and you'll give up on it entirely before too long. That's why I highly recommend you take the easy road and invest a couple of dollars in a macro app.

When it comes to tracking your calories and macros, it's important to be patient with yourself. You'll make mistakes at times, or you won't know the calories in a certain meal and that's ok. You have to stay calm and keep moving forward. When you get frustrated or rushed, you'll either quit or wrongly estimate how many calories are in what you're eating. And unfortunately, if you're not able to be diligent with tracking your calories and macros, you won't be successful with carb cycling.

The cool thing is that after a while, you'll get a good feel for how to you need to eat during your high and low carb days. You'll know approximately how much calories and macros are in the meals you're regularly eating. You can simply eyeball it and take an accurate guess as to how many calories are in the foods you're eating.

Of course this is something you'll acquire as time goes on with practice, so again remember that patience is the key! Initially though, tracking your macros can be frustrating at times if you've never done it before, so use the first couple of weeks as practice and a learning experience. The good news is that you don't need to be totally accurate down to the exact calorie when measuring. For example, if you need to eat 150 grams of protein one day, it's unlikely that you'll actually eat 150 grams spot on. That's completely ok; you want to get as close as you can, but don't go crazy trying to hit the numbers exactly. You want to largely be accurate and consistent for the long haul.

Chapter 11 Frequently Asked Questions

Can I Treat My High-Carb Days Like a Cheat Day?

No, you can't. There's a difference between a high-carb day and a cheat day. A cheat day brings with it the mentality that you can eat whatever you want whenever you want. This can make things get out of hand at times, causing you to overeat. A high-carb day, on the other hand, is a strategic part of the carb cycling process. You're still limited to eating a moderate amount of fat, and you'll want the majority of your carbs to come from quality food sources.

What if I'm not losing or gaining weight eating 13 calories per pound of bodyweight?

If you've been struggling to lose weight eating 13 calories per pound of bodyweight then I recommend using a different method to set your calories. Before I get into that though, you must first make sure you were actually eating 13 calories per pound of bodyweight minus 500 calories to lose 1 pound per week. It's easy to overestimate the amount of calories you're eating, and this could be the reason why you're not seeing results.

Once you've made sure you've accurately been tracking your calories, you can take your goal bodyweight, multiply it by 11 and then eat that many calories (don't subtract anything from the final calculated number).

Yes, I understand that your goal bodyweight will be a random number that you think you'll look good at, so take your best guess. Start on the higher side and work your way down from there if you still aren't losing weight.

Here's an example for a 250-pound male.

Current Weight 250

Goal Bodyweight 200

200 x 11= 2,200 daily calories

Let's say once this person reaches his goal of 200 pounds, he's still not satisfied with how he looks. From there, he can simply set a new goal bodyweight (i.e. 190 pounds for example) and go from there.

On the other hand, let's say you're struggling to add muscle eating 13 calories per pound of bodyweight plus 250 calories. Again, make sure you're accurately tracking the amount of calories you're eating. You could be miscounting your calories, and that would account for why you're not gaining any weight. Once you've made sure you're tracking things accurately, you can add 100 calories to your total resting metabolic rate weekly until you start gaining weight. For example:

A 180-pound male looking to gain weight would multiply his bodyweight by 13 to determine his maintenance calories.

180 x 13= 2,340

This person would then add 250 calories to 2,340 and get a total of 2,590 calories per day. If he eats 2,590 calories on a daily basis, he should start to gain 0.5 pound per week. However, if he doesn't, he can simply add 100 calories to his original 2,590 calories on a weekly basis until he does.

For example, on week 1, he would eat 2,690 calories. If he didn't gain any weight by the end of the week, he would eat 2,790 calories for the following week, and so on and so forth until he starts gaining weight.

What if I hit a plateau and I stop losing weight at my regular pace?

Let's say you've been losing weight just fine, but then all of the sudden you hit a wall and stop losing weight. In this case, take your new current bodyweight (which should be a lower number from when you first started) and multiply that by 13.

Take that number and subtract 250 from it. This will be your new daily caloric intake for you to lose weight.

This will have you losing weight at a rate of approximately 0.5 pound per week. You may have previously been losing weight at a rate of 1 pound per week, but now you'll lose at a rate of 0.5 pound per week.

This is because I don't want you to drastically reduce your calories all of the sudden, and because if you've hit a plateau, you're likely very close to hitting your goal weight anyway.

How many meals should I eat per day?

You can eat as many meals as you like throughout the day. Meal frequency doesn't matter for weight loss (16), but the total amount of calories you eat does. So eat however is easiest for you and your schedule.

I, myself, prefer to eat 3 meals a day and that works great for most people. However, feel free to eat 6 times per day or even as little as once per day. As long as you're hitting your macros, you'll be fine.

What do I do once I reach my goal bodyweight?

Contrary to what you might be thinking, things aren't going to be that much different from what you've been doing to lose weight. You still need to do flexible dieting and continue eating in the same manner that you previously were. This means that you should still keep the same eating schedule and keep eating similar meals to the ones that you were eating to lose weight.

However, there's one difference between maintenance and creating a caloric deficit to lose weight. The difference is that you get to consume more calories! How many calories? Well, this is pretty easy to figure out as a matter of fact.

Step #1: Determine at what rate you were losing weight (i.e. 1 pound per week).

Step #2: Translate pounds lost per week into calories.
    0.5 pound lost per week= 250 calories
    1 pound lost per week= 500 calories
    1.5 pounds lost per week= 750 calories
    2 pounds lost per week= 1,000 calories, etc.

Step #3: Add in those additional calories to what you were previously eating to maintain your new weight.

For example, let's say someone was losing weight at a rate of 1 pound per week by eating 1,850 calories per day. Once he hits his goal weight, he needs to eat 2,350 calories (1,850+500) per day to maintain his new weight.

You'll also need to recalculate your macro percentages. Continuing with this example, this individual would need to do the following with his new caloric intake:

2,350 x .40= 940 daily calories from protein

2,350 x .35= 822.5 daily calories from carbs
2,350 x .25= 587.5 daily calories from fat

How much weight should I lift during the workouts?

Lift as much weight as you possibly can for the given rep range. Initially, you won't know how much weight to use, so you'll have to take your best guess. For example, let's say you're doing bench press for 8 reps. You think you can lift around 150 pounds for that many reps, but on your first set, you easily complete 10 reps.

This means the weight is too light and you need to increase it for the next set. On the next set, you lift 165 pounds and struggle to complete the 8th rep. This is what you want to happen, and it means you've found a good weight to use. Once you can complete all 3 sets for 8 reps with 165 pounds, move up to 170 the next time you bench press. If you can't complete 8 reps for all 3 sets, stick with 165 until you can. Here's an example:

Workout 1: Bench Press with 165 pounds
Set 1: 8 reps
Set 2: 8 reps
Set 3: 7 reps

Because you only completed 7 reps on the last set, stick with 165 for the next workout.

Workout 2: Bench Press with 165 pounds
Set 1: 8 reps
Set 2: 8 reps
Set 3: 8 reps

Because you completed all 3 sets for 8 reps, move up to 170 on your next workout with bench press.

Note: It's better to use a weight that's too heavy and miss a rep or two than it is to use a weight that's too light and leave some reps in the tank. For example, it's better to do 170 pounds and only complete 6 reps instead of 8 as opposed to using 155 pounds and stopping at 8 reps even though you could've easily done more reps.

How Fast Should I Lose Weight?

The more weight you have to lose, the faster the rate at which you can lose the weight. For example, if you have 50+ pounds to lose, you can lose weight at a rate of 2 pounds or more per week. If you only have 5 pounds to lose, then lose weight at a rate of 0.5 pound per week.

For most people, losing 1 pound per week is the sweet spot. You'll be creating an average caloric deficit of 500 calories daily. At this pace, you'll be losing weight fairly quickly, and you won't be miserable all of the time from a complete lack of calories.

How much water should I drink on a daily basis?

Your body is made up of about 60% water, so it's important to consume water for several reasons. Drinking water regularly:

- Helps keep your joints and ligaments fluid, which can help prevent injury
- Helps control your caloric intake
- Flushes out toxins
- Improves skin quality
- Improves kidney function
- Improves your focus

Many people recommend that you should drink 1 gallon of water per day. This is a blanket answer that doesn't meet individual needs. This recommendation would have a 100-pound woman drinking the same amount of water as a 200-pound man. Absurd!

Other health experts advise drinking eight 8-ounce glasses (64 ounces total) of water a day. But again 64 ounces isn't going to be enough for most people. What should you do then? I don't keep track of my water intake—I go by how I feel and the color of my urine.

Your body's own thirst mechanism will be accurate in telling you if you need more water. If you feel thirsty, go drink some water. If not, you're probably ok. You can also use the color of your urine to judge how hydrated you are. If your urine is yellow, then you should drink more water. If it's clear then you should be good to go. This keeps things simple and it's one less thing you have to keep track of.

Are there any supplements that you recommend I take?

Most supplements are a complete waste of money. There's not a single supplement that's required in order for you to build muscle or burn fat. In fact, I advise for the first 6 weeks of your IIFYM diet that you don't take *any* supplements at all.

This is because I want you to see for yourself that it really is possible for you to get results without supplements. Your hard work and dedication matter way more than any pill or powder.

With that being said, there are a few supplements I recommend if you have the budget for them:

#1: Protein Powder:

You can't have a recommended list of supplements without protein powder on the list, right? Just kidding. But this has to be one of the most overhyped supplements of all time.

I think that the media does a really good job of making us believe that we must take protein powder to build muscle or take it to prevent muscle loss. I do think that protein powder can provide some benefits if *you need it*.

If you struggle to consistently hit your macros with protein then I would consider investing in a protein powder. Protein is necessary to help build and prevent the breakdown of muscle.

Therefore, ensuring that your muscle is spared is a good thing. However, don't go out of your way and eat more calories just for the sake of consuming more protein.

#2: Fish/Krill Oil

These oils are great sources of Omega-3 fatty acids. This is a good thing because most people consume too many Omega-6 fatty acids with foods like vegetable and canola oil.

Ideally, you want to be consuming a 1 to 1 ratio of Omega-3's to Omega-6's. Fish and krill oil can help you narrow the gap between the two types of fatty acids that you're consuming.

The main benefit from consuming these oils is that they act as an anti-inflammatory in your body. When you consume Omega-6's on the other hand, they act as an inflammatory.

That's why it's important to strike a balance with both of the fatty acids. The anti-inflammatory benefit is great because it can reduce your risk of developing heart disease or high blood pressure.

Finally, reducing inflammation can aid in muscle recovery. If you're going to invest in fish or krill oil, make sure that it's a very high-grade supplement.

The way that some of the lower quality oils are processed inhibits the absorption of them, which would make them completely useless. As for investing in fish or krill oil, taking either one is fine really.

Krill oil does contain the antioxidant astaxanthin (17), which helps with joint health, boosts cognitive function and helps promote a healthy cholesterol balance, while fish oil does not. However, I have noticed that krill oil can be harder to find, and it's typically more expensive so don't sweat not buying it.

#3: Digestive Enzymes

This is my favorite supplement of all time, and it's probably one of the most underrated supplements as well. If your body can't absorb the vitamins and nutrients that you're consuming then what's the point?

The sad fact of the matter is that when our foods get cooked, many of the enzymes get destroyed. Digestive enzymes will not only help to replenish those enzymes missed from cooked foods, but it will also help your body to better break down and utilize the nutrients that you're eating.

Also, if you ever suffer regularly from bloating, heartburn or have bad skin, give digestive enzymes a try and see if you notice a difference. Of course, it's important to note that these enzymes need to be high quality if you want them to be of any use.

Simply going to the local grocery store and purchasing a $10 bottle of enzymes isn't going to cut it. You must buy a high-quality enzyme if you want to get any use out of it. Personally, I recommend using Bio Trust.

How Do I Motivate Myself to Go to the Gym?

Finding the motivation to go to the gym or eat right can be hard. No matter who you are, there will be times when you don't feel like working out. Having that feeling is ok, but you can't let it control you. There will be times when you'll have to do it anyway even when you don't feel like it.

That's what will ultimately separate a long-term successful fitness journey from failing at it. I do have some tips to help you out along the way:

Tip #1: Focus on Gradual Improvements

Many people make fitness an all-or-nothing game. They tell themselves that they'll workout 5 days a week and eat clean 100% of the time for the rest of their lives. Let's say you workout only 4 days one week. Are you a failure?

Of course not! You still worked out 4 days, but in your mind you are because you failed to reach 5 workouts. You make it hard to celebrate any small successes that you do have because the standards are too high.

Instead, focus on making smaller, more gradual improvements and celebrate any successes you have along the way. For example, start off with a goal to only workout 2 days per week if it's been years since you've last worked out. Once you achieve that goal, you'll feel good about yourself then you can move up to working out 3 days per week and so on.

Tip #2: Action Leads Motivation

People think they have to get the inspiration or motivation from somewhere in order to take the action necessary to workout. The reverse of that is actually true. You need to start by taking an action no matter how small. And once you get started, you'll likely want to continue on with what you're doing.

When I think about everything I have to do to workout such as put my gym clothes on, drive to the gym, workout with a bunch of grueling exercises, drive back and shower, I start to make up silly excuses as to why I should skip this time. Instead, I'll tell myself to do just one exercise when I get to the gym and not pressure myself to do anything more. After I finish that first exercise, it's always easier for me to finish the rest of the workout.

You just have to get started. Try this out for any healthy habit you want to start. For example, if you want to start flossing your teeth, tell yourself you'll only floss one tooth and don't pressure yourself to do anything more than that!

Tip #3: Put Your Own Money on the Line

Money is a very powerful motivator. And you can use your own money to motivate yourself to start working out more. Here's what you're going to do—give someone a good amount of money. Not $20, but something that would actually hurt you—$100, $200, $500, or whatever you can't afford to lose.

Then tell your friend that if you don't go to the gym 3 days this week, for example, they get to keep the money. When you give up the money in the first place, you'll fight to get it back. This is much different than telling yourself you'll give the money to someone after you miss your workouts.

It's too easy to make an excuse and not give away the money. Give the money up in the first place and make sure your friend actually holds you accountable to it. This is by far the best way to get motivation to workout. There's a real cost involved if you don't comply. You'll either get ripped or go broke trying.

Conclusion

Thanks for getting this book and reading it all the way through to the end! Carb cycling is a good way to get and stay in shape for the rest of your life. You simply have to stay dedicated. Carb cycling works as long as you put forth the effort needed.

Feel free to email me at thomas@rohmerfitness.com with any fitness questions you may have.

And finally, if this book was helpful, please take a few minutes and leave a review. Your feedback will help me make better content for you in the future!

Sources

(1) https://www.ncbi.nlm.nih.gov/pubmed/8697046

(2) http://ajcn.nutrition.org/content/early/2013/06/26/ajcn.113.064113.abstract

(3) https://www.ncbi.nlm.nih.gov/pmc/articles/PMC3419346/

(4) https://www.ncbi.nlm.nih.gov/pubmed/16918875

(5) https://www.ncbi.nlm.nih.gov/pubmed/16320856

(6) http://circ.ahajournals.org/content/106/4/523.full

(7) https://www.hindawi.com/journals/isrn/2013/435027/

(8) https://www.ncbi.nlm.nih.gov/pubmed/19927027

(9) https://www.ncbi.nlm.nih.gov/pmc/articles/PMC4213385/

(10) https://www.ncbi.nlm.nih.gov/pubmed/19935843

(11) https://www.ncbi.nlm.nih.gov/pmc/articles/PMC3381813/

(12) http://www.ncbi.nlm.nih.gov/pubmed/18197184

(13) http://www.ncbi.nlm.nih.gov/pubmed/20473222

(14) http://www.health.harvard.edu/newsletter_article/Walking-Your-steps-to-health

(15) https://www.ncbi.nlm.nih.gov/pubmed/18787373

*Recipes courtesy of users at sparkpeople.com

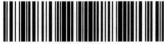

Made in the USA
Columbia, SC
19 April 2018